Mara Ilka H. de Medeiros Batista
Marcília Ribeiro Paulino
Alessandra de A. Tavares Carvalho

Oral health in a women's prison unit

Mara Ilka H. de Medeiros Batista
Marcília Ribeiro Paulino
Alessandra de A. Tavares Carvalho

Oral health in a women's prison unit

Experience of caries in male and female prison guards

ScienciaScripts

Imprint
Any brand names and product names mentioned in this book are subject to trademark, brand or patent protection and are trademarks or registered trademarks of their respective holders. The use of brand names, product names, common names, trade names, product descriptions etc. even without a particular marking in this work is in no way to be construed to mean that such names may be regarded as unrestricted in respect of trademark and brand protection legislation and could thus be used by anyone.

Cover image: www.ingimage.com

This book is a translation from the original published under ISBN 978-613-9-66220-3.

Publisher:
Sciencia Scripts
is a trademark of
Dodo Books Indian Ocean Ltd. and OmniScriptum S.R.L publishing group

120 High Road, East Finchley, London, N2 9ED, United Kingdom
Str. Armeneasca 28/1, office 1, Chisinau MD-2012, Republic of Moldova, Europe
Printed at: see last page
ISBN: 978-620-7-99481-6

SUMMARY

CHAPTER 1

INITIAL CONSIDERATIONS ON BIOFILM, ENDODONTIC TREATMENT AND HERBAL MEDICINE

CARLUS ALBERTO OLIVEIRA DOS SANTOS;
KAROLYNE DE MELO SOARES;
APARECIDA THARLLA LEITE DE CALDAS;
MARIA REGINA MACÊDO-COSTA.

Microorganisms in their organised form (consortium) are responsible for causing and perpetuating most oral diseases. A heterogeneous composition of micro-organisms (MO), including those considered super-infectious and commonly associated with opportunistic and persistent infections, such as enteric micro-organisms, pseudomonads, staphylococci and yeasts, can easily be found in the root canal system. In endodontics, these infectious agents are responsible for the development of necrotic pulps, periapical pathology and post-treatment root canal diseases (MACÊDO- COSTA; SANTOS et al., 2018; ALAGL et al., 2017; SIQUEIRA JÚNIOR, 2003).

Although mechanical instrumentation is one of the most important steps in root canal treatment, and no matter how flexible the instruments used in endodontic practice are, they are unable to enter the branches of the root canal and sanctify them, requiring the use of chemical aids (SQAs) for microbial eradication and neutralisation of their products during endodontic treatment (GUNESER et al., 2016).

Various substances can be applied during the chemical-mechanical preparation of root canals; however, most of these substances have undesirable effects when used inadvertently. Toxicity to periapical tissues, hypersensitivity reactions and microbial resistance are adverse reactions inherent to sodium hypochlorite (NaOCl) and/or chlorhexidine digluconate (DCLX), for example (SIQUEIRA JÚNIOR, 2001; FERRETI et al., 2011).

NaOCl has been used as an endodontic irrigant for more than four decades.

Although it has excellent antimicrobial action and is an excellent tissue solvent, in high concentrations it is toxic to periapical tissues (VARISE et al., 2014; MOHAMMADI et al., 2013). Other risks may be associated with NaOCL, such as: emphysema, allergy, carcinogenic effect, offensive odour and taste; and also failure to remove the smearley layer which acts as a gateway for bacterial entry and multiplication. The effectiveness of DCLX is unquestionable, however, this SQA can cause microbial resistance, tooth staining, taste interference and studies have reported negative effects on cellular compounds (MICHELOTTO et al., 2008; OZAN et al., 2007; ALMEIDA et al., 2014; ALAGL et al., 2017).

Considering the increase in the occurrence of persistent or refractory endodontic infections related to superinfecting microorganisms in the oral environment, and the absence of a totally effective and safe auxiliary chemical substance, the development of alternative and economically viable natural solutions to replace commonly used antimicrobials is required (ALAGL et al., 2017; GUNESER et al., 2016).

An attractive source for these requirements is plant extracts, since they have a wide molecular diversity and greater safety than products derived from chemical synthesis. In addition, the popular acceptance of herbal medicine has reinforced the importance of more studies in this area, in order to introduce only those products proven to be effective and safe onto the market (COUTINHO et al., 2008; SILVA et al., 2007; LEITÃO et al., 2006).

Brazil has an enormous biodiversity, including several plants of economic interest (ALBUQUERQUE et al., 2007). The North and Northeast regions of the country are the ones that concentrate most of the existing plants, which allows access to numerous types of plants and fruit species (MATTIETTO; LOPES; MENEZES, 2010; MOREIRA et al., 2002).

Among these plants, **Spondias mombin**, popularly **known as "cajá", belongs to the** *Anacardiaceae* family. *The* leaves are used to gargle, as an astringent, in inflammations of the mouth and throat. There are reports of its use in the mouth in cases of prostatitis and cold sores. As far as biological activities are concerned, the following have been cited: antimicrobial and antioxidant activity (CORTHOUT et al. 1994; ABO et al.,

1999; SILVA et al. 2012) antiviral (SILVA et al. 2011); leishmanicidal (ACCIOLY, 2001).

The aim of this book was to clarify the main factors related to endodontic infections, as well as the use of herbal medicine in dentistry. It is a work carried out through an analytical review of the relevant literature.

CHAPTER 2

DENTAL TISSUES, ENDODONTIC TREATMENT AND INTERNAL DENTAL ANATOMY.

CARLUS ALBERTO OLIVEIRA DOS SANTOS;
KAROLYNE DE MELO SOARES;
MARIA REGINA MACÊDO-COSTA

From a histological point of view, the dental pulp is a loose, innervated and vascularised connective tissue responsible for dentin formation and enamel and dentin nutrition. Because it has great repair potential, pulp necrosis only occurs when tissue repair mechanisms fail (LEONARDI et al., 2011).

Dentin is a calcified connective tissue made up of millions of canaliculi. Dentinal tubules have an important relationship with dentin sensitivity, as they extend from the dentin-amel junction to the pulp. They act as transfer routes for stimuli and irritants to the pulp tissue, which is explained by the hydrodynamic theory (RIBEIRO et al., 2012; VOGTMANN et al., 2016).

The dental pulp is responsible for tooth vitality and has a number of functions, including sensory, formative, nutritive and defensive, constituting a complex organ protected from external agents by dentin, enamel, alveolar bone, cementum and periodontal ligament. However, patients who are affected by periodontal diseases caused or intensified by smoking require sub or supragingival scraping, making them more susceptible to infections due to the removal of the cementum and subsequent exposure of the dentinal tubules (LEITÃO et al., 2006).

The pathogens generate inflammatory responses that induce a reduction in vascular reactivity and vasodilation, aggregation of red blood cells and an increase in blood viscosity, which consequently leads to major pulp involvement, which usually requires more radical pulp treatment (RIBEIRO et al., 2012).

Endodontics is known as the speciality of dentistry that studies periradicular tissues and the morphology, pathology and physiology of the dental pulp. This area of practice for dental surgeons is part of the basic curriculum of dentistry courses in Brazil and studies diseases and injuries to the pulp and associated periradicular conditions, as well as the biology of the normal pulp, its aetiology, diagnosis and prevention (BRITO, 2016; DA CONCEIÇÃO et al., 2012).

Root canal treatment basically consists of accessing the root canals to remove the pulp tissue, which may be inflamed or necrotic, cleaning and shaping the canals, and then filling them with an inert, biocompatible, dimensionally stable material that allows the health of the periapical region to regenerate (LEITÃO et al., 2006).

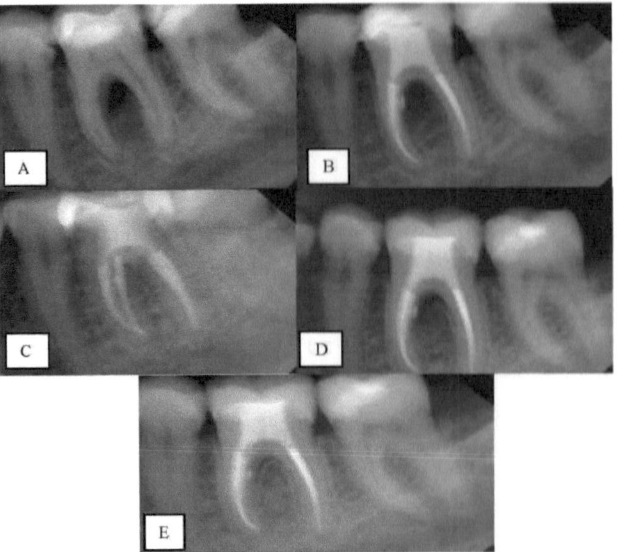

Figure 1 - Root canal treatment in a case of apical and inter-root (furcation) pathology. A) Pre-treatment radiograph of tooth 36 shows an inter-radicular lesion. B-C) Post-treatment radiographs after root canal preparation and obturation. D-E) Two-month control radiograph suggests rapid repair.

Source: Hargreaves; Cohen, 2011.

Endodontics is indicated in various cases to maintain the function of the dental unit in the oral cavity, ranging from phonation and aesthetics to mastication. Treatment of the root canal system (RCS) may be indicated when there has been major destruction of the tooth's crown to the point of exposing the pulp chamber as a result of a caries lesion or even mechanical trauma leading to crown fracture. There are also endodontic treatments indicated for orthodontic trauma and endo-periodontal lesions (LEITÃO et al., 2006; CHEN et al., 2016; GOMES et al., 1997).

Internal anatomy of the root canal

From a morphological point of view, teeth have individual characteristics, both externally and internally. Knowledge of these characteristics is of great relevance to dental practice, as it is known that many of the mishaps encountered during dental care arise due to the existence of anatomical variations and these have repercussions on the specialities of dentistry, such as endodontics (SIQUEIRA JÚNIOR, 2001).

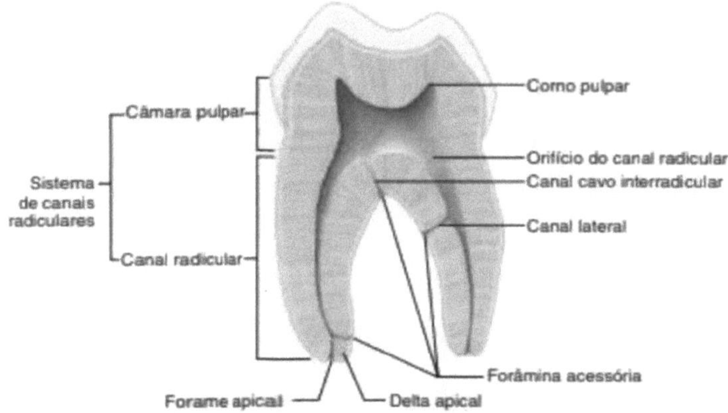

Figure 2 - Main anatomical components of root canals.

Source: Hargreaves; Cohen, 2011.

Studies involving dental anatomy are not new. The anatomy of root canals has been the subject of studies since 1942, and despite the many observations described by various authors in their works, there are still doubts about the internal and external morphological aspects of various groups of teeth (SCAINE et al., 2005).

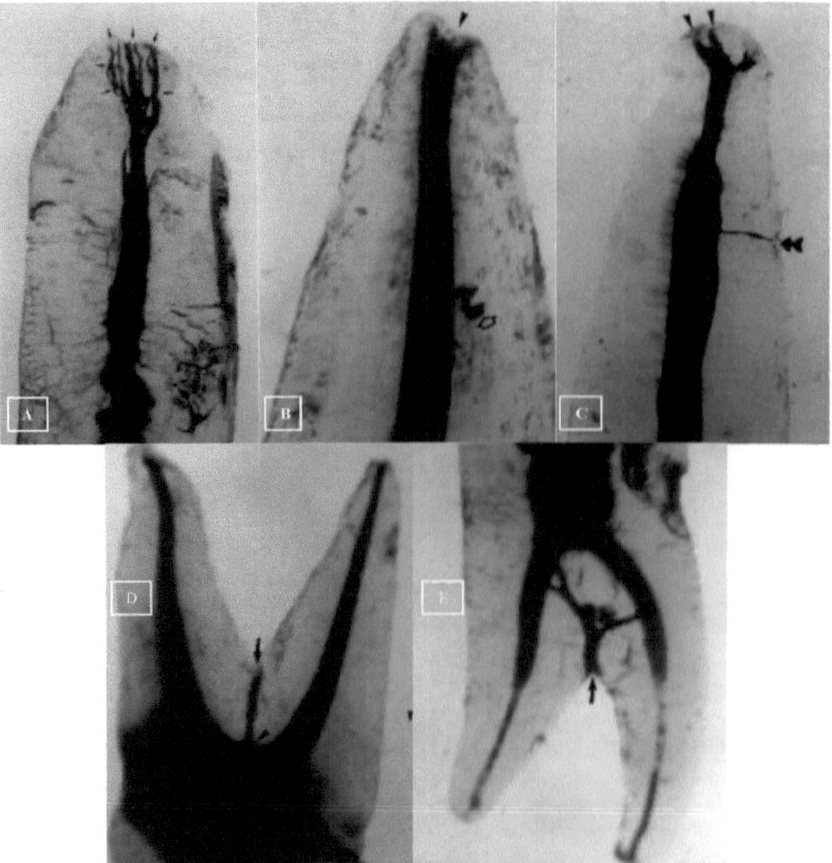

Figure 3 - A-B-C-D) Anatomical variation in root canals of different maxillary lateral incisors, with a proximal view, through macroscopic sections and diaphanisation. E) Proximal view of the root canals of a biradicular maxillary lateral incisor, diaphanised and also through macroscopic sections, where anatomical variation can also be seen.

Source: Azeredo et al., 2005.

Santos et al. (2010) state that SCR is still considered a mystery to be unravelled, as there may be countless anatomical variations that need to be clarified so that the clinician can interpret and develop their role properly, even if the endodontist is experienced. Thus, unusual situations can surprise the endodontist in terms of the individual characteristics of dental groups. It is therefore necessary to recognise the possible anatomical variations, thereby reducing the risk of unsuccessful endodontic therapy.

Dental elements are similar to each other, but variations are visible from one element to another within the same dental group. As one of the most important teeth in endodontics, the maxillary first molar has undoubtedly been one of the most researched and investigated elements, with the aim of increasing clinical success in endodontic treatment (BURNS; HERBRANSON, 2000).

Faced with this morphological complexity, which can compromise the success of endodontic treatment, various techniques can be used to overcome these obstacles. Radiographic examination, for example, should be carried out prior to endodontic therapy, helping to identify the anatomy of the tooth to be treated. Despite their effectiveness, conventional radiographic examinations have some limitations, such as radiographic overlaps; therefore, after coronal access, with a thorough inspection of the pulp chamber floor, we can be more certain of the total number of canals in the tooth in question (MANCILHA et al., 2007; RENNER, 2005).

According to White and Pharoah (2000), radiographic examinations are particularly useful in assessing the following points:

a) amount of bone present;

b) condition of the alveolar ridge;

c) bone loss in the furcation region;

d) width of the periodontal ligament space; 12

e) local factors that intensify periodontal disease such as: dental calculus, poor adaptation of dental restorations, excessive restorations;

f) root length and morphology, as well as the crown-root ratio;

g) anatomical conditions such as: position of the maxillary sinus in relation to periodontal destruction, presence of supernumerary teeth, 1mpacted teeth or tooth agenesis; and

h) pathological conditions: caries, periapical lesions, root resorption.

Technology is in favour of endodontics. Making use of technological devices can help the endodontist during root canal treatment. With the advent of microscopy in endodontics, the localisation - and consequently quantification - of root canals present on the floor of a pulp chamber has become an easier and safer procedure when compared to the detection of root canal entry holes with the naked eye or with the aid of magnifying glasses (SANTOS et al., 2010; KATO et al., 2016).

The use of a clinical microscope was introduced in endodontics to magnify and illuminate the operative field. This feature favours the visualisation of details, enabling the dental surgeon to remove dentin more selectively, minimising errors. Many studies show that this artefact significantly increases the chance of locating canals (RENNER, 2005).

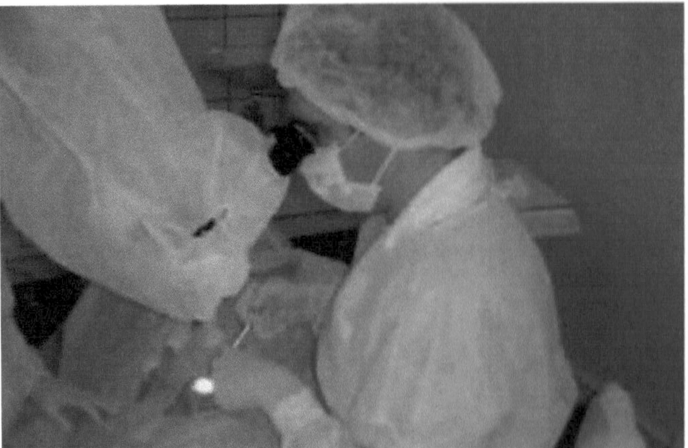

Figure 4 - Clinical procedure carried out with the aid of a clinical microscope for endodontic treatment.

Source: Souza-Filho; Soares, 2018.

Another factor that can help determine the number of canals or branches present in root canals is the use of stainless steel instruments with pre-curvatures, which can provide a clinical procedure capable of informing the internal anatomy of root canals three-dimensionally (LOPES et al., 2010).

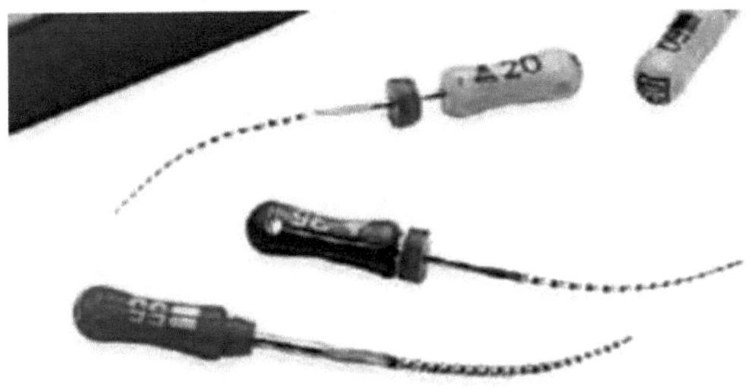

Figura 5 - Stainless steel instrument.

Source: Reis, 2015.

Internally, the root canal has various configurations which, as described above, can have different characteristics depending on the tooth group. A very important structure that must be considered in endodontic treatment is the canal-dentin-cementum boundary (CDC) or apical constriction, which represents the point of greatest constriction of the root canal, since the canal is represented by two cones joined by their vertices where one of the cones represents the dentin canal and the other the cementum canal (RENNER, 2005).

Apical constriction not only limits the pulp cavity, but also outlines the extent to which the host's organic defences are actually effective against the progression of bacterial etiological agents (MONTEIRO, 2016; SANTOS et al., 2010; LOPES et al., 2010).

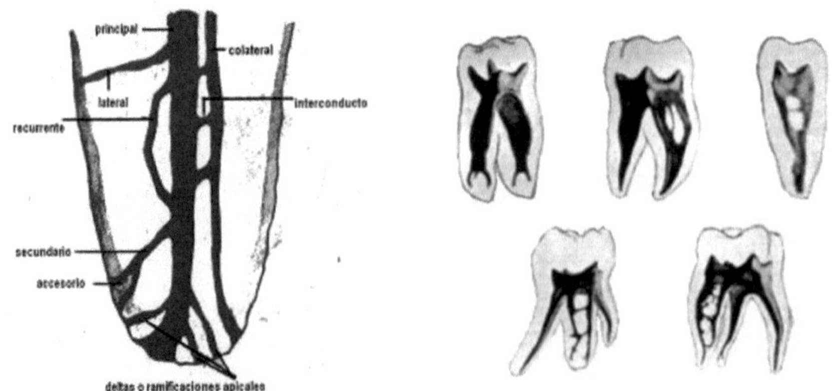

Figura 6 - Root canal branching in the apical third.

Source: Rodrígez, 2017.

CHAPTER 3

MICROBIOLOGICAL ASPECTS OF ENDODONTIC INFECTIONS

CARLUS ALBERTO OLIVEIRA DOS SANTOS;
KAROLYNE DE MELO SOARES;
MARIA REGINA MACÊDO-COSTA.

The various branches and dentinal tubules present in the SCR make the root canal environment favourable for the adhesion of pathogenic microorganisms. Microorganisms present in the SCR have been shown to be the main cause of endodontic therapy failure, both due to their metabolic products and the effect of biofilm that can colonise accessory canals, isthmuses, apical deltas and dentinal tubules, making it difficult to eliminate them through instrumentation, the use of irrigating substances and intracanal medication (MONTEIRO, 2016; DA CONCEIÇÃO et al., 2012).

It is estimated that in coronal dentin there are 20,000 dentinal tubules per m2 near the enamel and 45,000 tubules per m2 near the pulp tissue. This peculiarity of dentin tissue is responsible for its highly permeable characteristics and dentin exposure represents the main access route for bacteria and their by-products to reach the pulp cavity, since the diameter of dentin tubules is entirely compatible with that of most bacteria found in the oral cavity. However, the speed of bacterial invasion via dentinal tubules is directly related to the condition of the pulp tissue (PASSOS, 2014).

The area of dentin occupied by the canaliculi is 1% at the dentin-amel junction, increasing to 45% as it approaches the pulp chamber. The clinical implications of this data are enormous, because as the dentin is exposed in depth, its permeability increases, making the pulp more susceptible to chemical and bacterial irritants (LOPES et al., 2010).

The bacteria present in endodontic infections are only a restricted group of species from the total oral microbiota. Some bacteria need carbohydrates for energy. Certain conditions present in the root canal system allow anaerobic bacteria to grow

(OROZCO, 2016). Since there is a strong relationship between the species present in the root canal based on nutritional demand, the pathogenicity generated by the polymicrobial community depends on their synergism (SUNDQVIST, 1992; OROZCO, 2016).

Bacterial interactions arise from the needs of the food chain, in which the metabolism of some species produces the essential nutrients for the development of others (LOPES et al., 2010; PAISANO et al., 2010; OROZCO, 2016; TANOMARU-FILHO et al., 2006).

Sassone et al. (2007) assessed the composition of the microbiota present in the primary endodontic lesions of 111 single-rooted teeth with pulp necrosis. The samples were collected using sterile paper tips and analysed using the checkerboard test and PCR, obtaining a reading of 40 different bacterial species, the average of which reflected a number of around 22 species in each sample. **Enterococcus faecalis (89.3%), Campylobacter gracilis (89.3%), Leptotrichia buccalis (89.3%), Neisseria mucosa (87.5%), Prevotella melaninogenica (86.6%), Fusobacterium nucleatum ssp. vincentii (85.7%), Eubacterium saburreum (75.9%), Streptococcus anginosus (75%),** and **Veillonella parvula** (74.1%) were the most prevalent species.

Enterococcus faecalis is able to organise itself in the form of a biofilm, making it more resistant to phagocytosis, antibodies and antibiotics when compared to non-biofilm-forming organisms. It is a Gram-positive, facultative anaerobic bacterium, normally found in the gastrointestinal tract of humans and other mammals (ALVES et al., 2015). This microorganism also has several virulence factors such as lipoteichoic acid (LTA), peptidoglycan, cytolysin and aggregation substances, capable of inducing periapical inflammation (VASCONCELOS, 2016; LEE; BAEK, 2012).

Studies by Narayanan; Vaishnavi et al. (2010) showed that the most resistant strains already identified in endodontic infections include **Fusobacterium nucleatum, Prevotella spp., Campylobacter rectus, Streptococci (Streptococcus mitis, Streptococcus gordonii, Streptococcus anginosus, Streptococcus oralis), Lactobacilli (Lactobacillus paracasei and Lactobacillus acidophilus), Staphylococci, E. faecalis, Olsenella uli, Parvimonas micra, Pseudoramibacter alactolyticus, Propionibacterium spp, Actinomyces spp., Bifidobacterium**

spp. and Eubacterium spp.

Most Gram-negative bacteria, common in infected and untreated root canals, are more easily eliminated after chemical-mechanical preparation (CMP) followed or not by intracanal medication, usually based on calcium hydroxide. However, facultative or strict anaerobic Gram-positive bacteria have been isolated or detected in samples taken for studies after endodontic treatment. These findings suggest that Gram-positive bacteria have greater resistance and adaptability to the environmental conditions of instrumented and often medicated root canals (WERLANG et al., 2016; SIQUEIRA JÚNIOR; RÔÇAS, 2014).

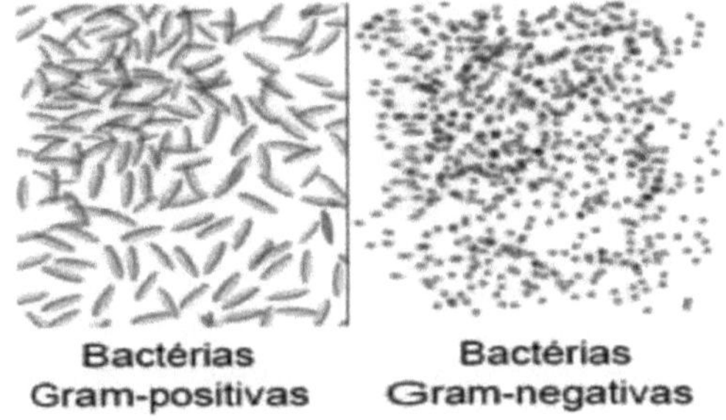

Figura 7 - Gram-positive and gram-negative bacteria.

Source: AbcMed, 2018.

With the capacity for microbial resistance, several studies have been carried out in an attempt to obtain a drug that eliminates bacteria or inactivates their endotoxins in teeth with chronic periapical lesions. Although chemical-mechanical treatment of infected root canals is effective in reducing root canal infection, viable microorganisms are often isolated after treatment. Some authors have reported the importance of cleaning with suitable substances and/or instruments to promote better pharmacological action of the drugs used in dressings and/or intracanal fillings, offering conditions for a faster and more organised organic response. Both single and multiple visit protocols are currently used to reduce the microbial content in canals (TRINCHES et al., 2014; TANOMURO-FILHO et al., 2010; DORNELLES et al., 2011).Another important microbial species that should be considered is **Staphylococcus aureus**, which is among the most resistant species found in infected root canals and is often associated with endodontic treatment failures (TRINCHES et al., 2014).

Chart 1 - Classification of micro-organisms in the types and subtypes of infections.

Primary infections		Persistent secondary infections	Extranadicular infections
Chronic perimyicular injury	Acute perinadicular abscess		
Bacteroides	*Porphyromonas*	*Enterococcus*	*Actinomyces*
Treponema	*Treponema*	*Actinomyces*	*Propionibacterium*
Prevotella	*Fusobacterium*	*Streptococcus*	
Porphyromonas	*Bacteroides*	*Condida*	
Fusobacteiium	*Prevotella*	*Propionibacterium*	
Peptostreptococcus	*Streptococcus*	*Staphylococcus*	
Streptococcus	*Pepiostreptococcus*	*Seudomonas*	
Eubacterium			
Actinomyces			
Campylobacter			
References*			

Source: Altamirano, 2017.

Enterococcus faecalis

Enterococcus faecalis is considered the most worrying micro-organism when it comes to persistent endodontic lesions. This characteristic is justified by its ability to resist endodontic treatment (resistance under unfavourable conditions) and, due to this ability, it has been used in various **in vitro** studies as a parameter for evaluating the effectiveness of antimicrobial procedures (NACIF et al., 2010; PARADELLA et al., 2007; ALEIXO et al., 2015).

The ability of the genus Enterococcus to form a biofilm allows it to colonise inert and biological surfaces, protect against antimicrobial agents and the action of phagocytes, mediating adhesion and invasion of host cells (DISTEL et al., 2002; ALVES et al., 2013). Histologically, they appear as spherical or ovoid cells that can occur in pairs or short chains in liquid media, when united they form whitish colonies with a creamy appearance (PORTENIER; WALTIMO; HAAPASALO, 2003).

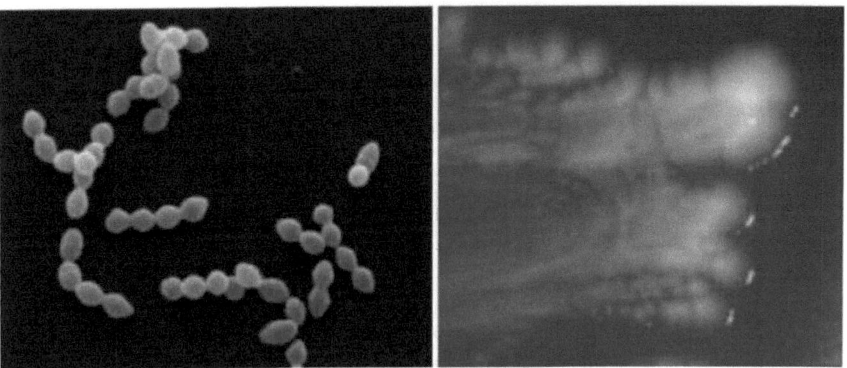

Figure 8 - Cells (scanning electron micrograph) and colonies (blood agar plate) of **Enterococcus spp.**
Source: Portenier; Waltimo; Haapasalo, 2003.

According to Nacif et al. (2010) and Paradella et al. (2007), **E. faecalis** species are resistant to the antimicrobial effects of calcium hydroxide, probably due to the effective proton pumping system that maintains optimal cytoplasmic pH levels, making endodontic treatment difficult. This MO is still the most frequently isolated from teeth with post-endodontic treatment infections, and is a concern for clinicians. The isolation of **E. faecalis** from root canals is not related to the use of certain filling materials, but rather to its low sensitivity to microbial agents and its ability to inactivate them.

Table 1 - Results, in percentages, of the sensitivity and resistance to antimicrobials of 13 samples of **E. Faecalis.**

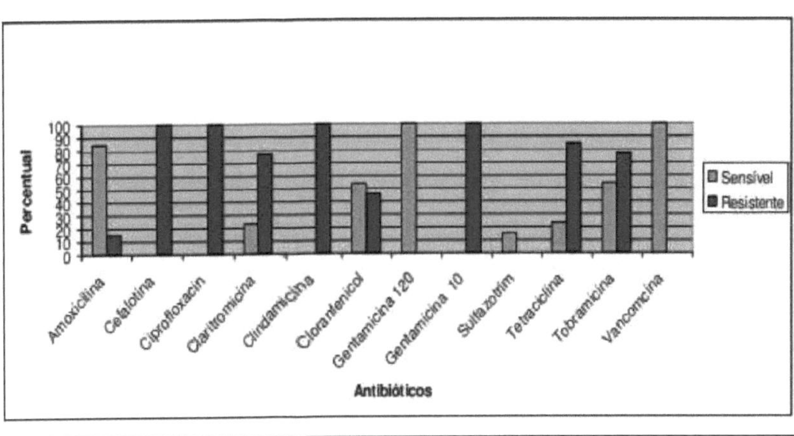

ANTIM1CR0BIAN0S	EVALUATION

	Sensitive		Resistant	
	N* of samples	%	N* of samples	%
Ainoxicillin	11	84.6	2	15,4
Cephalothin	0	0	13	100,0
Ciprofloxaem	0	0	13	100,0
Clarithromycin	3	23.0	10	77,0
Clindamycin	0	0	13	100,0
Chlorantemcol	7	53.8	6	46,2
Gentamicin 10	0	0	13	100,0
Gentamicin 120	13	100,0	0	0
Sulfazotrim	2	15,4	11	84,6
Tetracycline	3	23.0	10	77,0
Tobramycin	7	53.8	6	46,2
Vancomycin	13	100,0	0	0

Source: Pinto et al., 2011.

Most clinical cases show root canals infected with **E. faecalis** that have remained asymptomatic for years because they have not responded to conventional endodontic therapy and were discovered by periapical radiographs that revealed periapical lesions, often at an advanced stage. Some patients show mild pain and the process can worsen during endodontic treatment (OLANDER et al., 2003). In 81.5% of cases of teeth without lesions associated with the apex, strains of **E. Faecalis** can be isolated in recurrent pulp and periapical infections. This bacterial species prevents the release of hydrolytic enzymes by polymorphonucleated cells, which may explain its dominance in pulp infections (GOMES et al., 2008).

One of the greatest capabilities of **E. Faecalis** is its ability to resist unfavourable environments when exposed to bile salts, acid, heat, lack of glucose, sodium hypochlorite and when stored in tap water. Studies show that this OM can remain viable in root canals **in vitro** for a period of 12 months without additional nutrients.

Clinically, the ability of **E. faecalis** to resist and survive extended periods in limited nutritional environments represents an important characteristic of the pathogenesis of this species in pathological processes of endodontic treatment failure (SABETI et al., 2004; VIVACQUA-GOMES et al., 2005).

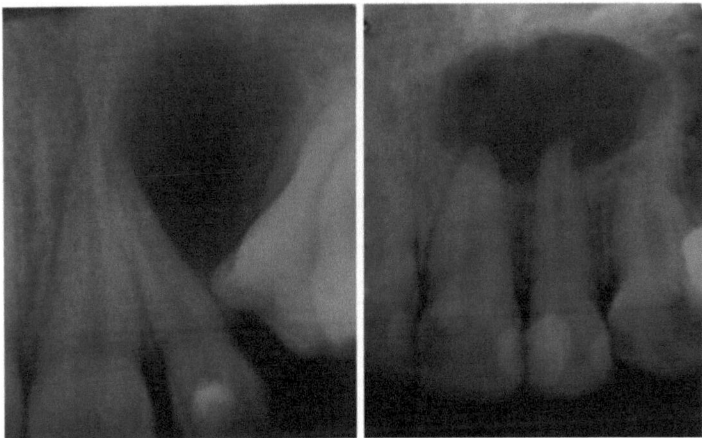

Figure 9 - Radiographically visible chronic periapical lesion.

Source: Lionardi et al., 2011.

Although **E. faecalis** are MOs that show marked microbial resistance, the mechanisms of resistance have not yet been fully clarified, however, the ease of transferring genes that code for the production of virulence factors: gelatinases, cytolysins, Enterococcus surface proteins, as well as Enterococcus aggregation substances, may account for this resistance in humans (VIVACQUA-GOMES et al., 2005).

E. faecalis are present in primary infections, but in small proportions. These OM are frequently found in endodontically filled canals with signs of chronic apical periodontitis, isolated in between 23% and 70% of positive cultures, and there may be several occurrences in monoculture (PINHEIRO et al., 2003; PARADELLA et al., 2007).

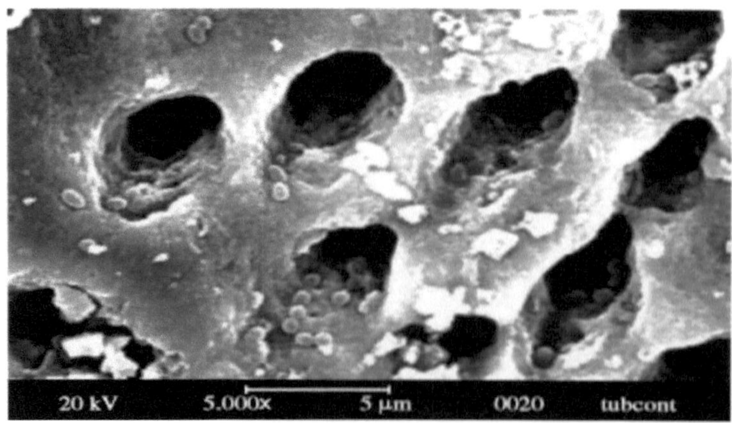

Figure 10 - Microscopic view of **Enterococus faecalis** in human dentin.

Source: Paradella et al., 2007.

Staphylococcus aureus

Conceptually, periapical lesions correspond to immunoinflammatory reactions, in which microorganisms and their by-products are considered the etiological agents of their development and dissipation. Their pathogenic capacity stems from pulp necrosis, since the mortified pulp makes a favourable environment for these bacteria to establish themselves (GOMES et al., 2008; PARADELLA et al., 2007).

Staphylococcus are the Gram-positive bacteria that most commonly produce betalactamases, inactivating penicillins. Various alterations to the structure of beta-lactam agents have been developed to protect the beta-lactam ring from enzymatic hydrolysis, increasing the effectiveness of the antibiotic in beta-lactamase-producing microorganisms (RÔÇAS, 2014; BRITO, 2016). The isoxazolyl-penicillins, which include oxacillin and dicloxacillin, are small-spectrum antibiotics that are resistant to beta-lactamases and are indicated almost exclusively for staphylococcal infections (BRITO, 2016).

Another important characteristic is that bacteria of the Staphylococcus genus are also capable of producing a wide variety of extracellular toxins and virulence factors, which are related to pathogenicity and mechanisms of resistance to available antimicrobials. These include toxic shock syndrome toxin 1 (TSST-1), recognised as the main cause of toxic shock syndrome (TSS) in humans, characterised by fever, hypotension, congestion in various organs and lethal shock (GOMES et al., 2008; PINHEIRO et al., 2003; WERLANG, 2016).

Several species of staphylococcus may be associated with dental abscesses, abscesses associated with osseointegrated implants and osteomyelitis (peri-implantitis) and other clinical problems. Several studies have reported the persistence of **Staphylococcus spp.** after root canal cleaning and they are also resistant to the antiseptics and disinfectants most commonly used in endodontics (PINHEIRO et al., 2003; MARTINHO et al., 2010). According to Pinheiro et al., 2003, **Staphylococcus aureus** is among the most resistant species found in infected root canals and is often.

Although the resistance mechanisms of all microorganisms are not yet fully understood, it is known that the microbiota of open canals, i.e. those exposed to the oral environment, is different from that of closed canals, where the bacterial composition is predominantly anaerobic, while in open canals, the microorganisms are basically facultative (CHUEH et al., 2003).

CHAPTER 4

FAILURE IN ENDODONTIC THERAPY

CARLUS ALBERTO OLIVEIRA DOS SANTOS;
KAROLYNE DE MELO SOARES;
MARIA REGINA MACÊDO-COSTA.

The failure of endodontic treatments is present in the clinical routine of the endodontist and raises doubts as to its etiology. For a satisfactory prognosis, the diagnosis must be carried out carefully and the signs and symptoms of the causes of endodontic failure must be investigated, so that an appropriate treatment plan can then be drawn up according to the aetiology of the case (WERLANG, 2016).

Endodontic failure can be defined as the inability of endodontic treatment to eliminate the microorganisms in the RCC, making this residual microbiota incompatible with the individual's state of health and making it impossible to repair the periradicular tissues, resulting in the existence of post-treatment periradicular lesions. These lesions are classified as: emergent (appeared after treatment), persistent (persisted after treatment) or recurrent (recurred after treatment) (LACERDA et al., 2016).

The failure of endodontic treatments has also been associated with the resistance of pathogenic microorganisms to the drugs used to combat them. This resistance mechanism results from physiological or structural changes in the bacterial cell, which represents a survival strategy against the abusive attack of antimicrobial agents (FORBES et al., 1998).

Studies have revealed a surprising increase in the antimicrobial resistance of bacteria that are commonly found in the root canals of teeth with endodontic infection. These bacteria have mechanisms that confer resistance to a variety of antibiotics commonly used in therapy (DI SANTI et al., 2015).

Table 2 - Interpretative values of the antimicrobials evaluated and classified as susceptible and resistant.

Antimicrobial agents	Susctivel	Resistant
Amoxicillin (AC)	≤8	≥16
Rifampidna < RJ)	≤1	≥4
Moxiiloxacma (MX)	≤2	≥8
Vancomidna (VA)	≤4	≥32
Tetradcline (TC)	≤4	≥16
CiproSoxadna (CI)	≤1	≥4
Chloramphenicol (CL)	≤8	≥32
Benzdpcnicillin (PG)	≤8	≥16
Amoxicilliru * Davulanic acid (XL)	≤8	≥16
Doxidcline (DC)	≤4	≥16
Erythromycin (EM)	≤0.5	≥8
Azithromycin (AZ)	≤2	≥8

Source: Di Santini et al., 2015.

Based on the literature, it was observed that the etiology of endodontic therapy failure has been associated with microbial factors (intraradicular and extraradicular infection - bacteria, fungi) and non-microbial factors (endogenous - true cysts; exogenous - foreign body reaction). In addition, other aetiological agents have been correlated as potential periradicular aggressors, such as the organism's defence response to instrumentation beyond the periapex, extrusion of irrigating liquid and overcrowding (LACERDA et al., 2016).

As previously mentioned, even after biomechanical preparation and obturation, bacterial biofilm can persist inside root canals (SIQUEIRA JÚNIOR; VERA et al., 2014; RÔÇAS, 2014; NAIR et al., 2005) and this persistence of microorganisms after treatment is the main cause of failure in endodontic therapy (SIQUEIRA, 2001).

The causes of failure are most often related to microbial factors and are didactically divided into persistent and secondary infection. In fact, these entities are not differentiated clinically, except in peculiar situations such as the appearance of lesions or acute periradicular abscesses in previously vital teeth. Faced with the possibility of therapy failure, endodontic professionals should have options at hand to increase the disinfection capacity of root canals, resulting in a higher percentage of successful cases (CHUEH et al., 2003).

Persistent infections

Persistent infection is infection that has persisted despite disinfection procedures and drastic changes to the microenvironment after the use of intracanal medications, irrigating substances and the action of mechanical instruments. Its aetiology is associated with both primary and secondary infection microorganisms. Persistent endodontic infections include post-treatment pulp and periapical infections, in which resistant enteric bacteria predominate (SIQUEIRA JÚNIOR; RÔÇAS, 2014).

Enterococcus faecalis is the most commonly isolated microorganism, especially in cases of conventional treatment failure, when retreatment is instituted. Although it can survive in alkaline pH, the exact pH for its elimination has not yet been determined (LACERDA et al., 2016; WERLANG et al., 2016; SIQUEIRA JÚNIOR; RÔÇAS, 2014).

Roças; Siqueira Júnior and Santos (2004) carried out a molecular study to determine possible associations between **Enterococcus faecalis** and different endodontic infections using 16S rDNA and PCR (Polymerase Chain Reaction). The samples were obtained from teeth with asymptomatic chronic apical periodontitis (n=21) - Group A; cases of acute apical periodontitis (n=10) - Group B; acute abscesses (n=19) - Group C; endodontically treated teeth with chronic periradicular lesions and no symptoms (n=30) - Group D. The species was detected in seven samples from G (A) (33.3%), one case from G (B) (10%), one of the exudates collected from G (C) (5.26%) and in 20 collections from G (D) (66.6%).

Statistical analysis revealed a higher prevalence of **E. faecalis** in chronic cases (without syntolaryngology) of initial endodontic treatments; the species was strongly associated with persistent periapical infections; and the average probability of **Enterococcus faecalis** being present in persistent infections resulting from the failure of the first treatment was 91 per cent. They evaluated endodontically treated teeth in a dental service in Taiwan and found that 70% of the cases, out of a total of 1085, had root canal fillings that were considered deficient (CHUEH et al., 2003).

Martinho et al. (2010) reported that the high antigenic activity of the bacterial endodontic content of primary root canal infection was a potent stimulus against macrophages in the release of IL-10 and TNF-a, demonstrating a positive correlation between the levels of endotoxins present in root canals and the production of IL-10 and TNF-a. However, little is known about endotoxins in persistent endodontic infection and their role in the development of clinical symptoms and destruction. In the study by Cardoso et al. (2016) culturable bacteria were detected in all root canal samples from teeth with persistent infection. However, there is controversy as to the origin of this type of infection, which results from persistent primary infection located in strategic areas not reached by instrumentation or from new infection of root systems by coronal leakage (secondary infection). Regardless, there is a consensus that the need for endodontic retreatment involves the elimination of apical periodontitis.

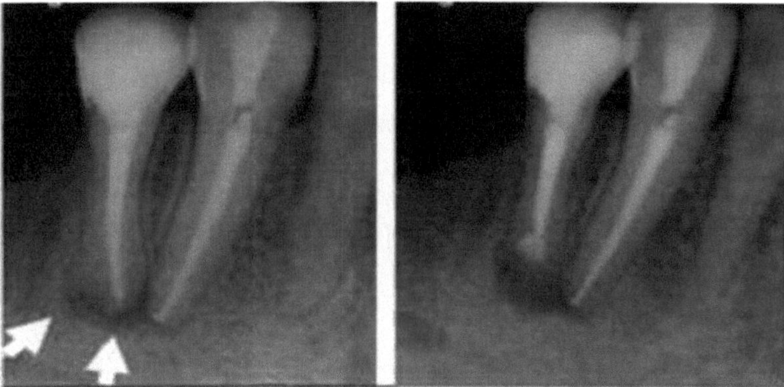

Figure 11- Radiographic examination of persistent endodontic infection causing bone resorption.

Source: Palmas, 2017.

CHAPTER 5

MAIN IRRIGATING AGENTS USED IN ENDODONTICS

CARLUS ALBERTO OLIVEIRA DOS SANTOS;
KAROLYNE DE MELO SOARES;
MARIA REGINA MACÊDO-COSTA.

An irrigating solution is considered essential in the preparation of the root canal for the sanitisation process, as it favours cleaning and shaping and neutralises necrotic content, which favours the enlargement of the root canal for subsequent filling (WEBER et al., 2003; PETREL et al., 2011).

As with all materials used in dental practice, certain minimum requirements must be met in order for them to be used safely. Thus, in order to effectively clean and disinfect the root canal system, the irrigant must be able to disinfect and penetrate the dentin and its tubules, offer a long-lasting antibacterial effect (substantivity), remove the smear layer and be antigenic, non-toxic or carcinogenic. Another capability of SQAS is that they must not have adverse effects on dentin, nor alter the three-dimensional sealing capacity of filling materials. Not least, the SQA must be low cost, easy to apply and not cause colour changes in the treated teeth. An ideal irrigating agent includes, in addition to the above, the ability to dissolve pulp tissue and inactivate endotoxins (CARDÉNAS et al., 2012; VINÍCIUS et al., 2011).

During chemical-mechanical preparation (CMP), chemical products are used in conjunction with mechanical instrumentation to reduce the bacterial load on dentinal tubules and root branches. Numerous chemical solutions are used in an attempt to sterilise root canals and the most effective and commonly used is sodium hypochlorite (NaOCl) in concentrations ranging from 1-6% (CARDÉNAS et al., 2012; ALTAMIRANO et al., 2017), 2017). Its unique ability to dissolve cellulose tissue and excellent antimicrobial potency makes it preferable to other irrigants such as 2% chlorohexidine solution (CHX) and calcium hydroxide [Ca(OH)], which have a varying degree of antimicrobial action. Several disadvantages of NaOCl have been cited previously, these include limited penetration into the complex canal system, toxicity, risk of emphysema, allergy, offensive odour and taste; and also failure to remove the smear layer which has been suggested as a gateway for bacterial entry and multiplication (ALTAMIRANO et al., 2017; PETREL et al., 2011).

Recent studies show that high concentrations of NaOCl can cause weakening of the dentin, decreasing its hardness and structural reliability, making the tooth susceptible to vertical fracture (VINÍCIUS et al., 2011),

Another irrigating agent widely used in endodontics is chlorhexidine digluconate (DCLX), which is less effective than NaOCl. DCLX is used effectively as a viable alternative to NaOCl, due to its broad antimicrobial spectrum of action, biocompatibility, but its disadvantage is that it can discolour the tooth and other problems reported as it can cause dryness and a burning sensation in the oral mucosa. Other studies show that DCLX can cause negative effects on cellular components (MICHELOTTO et al., 2008; WEBER et al., 2003).

The mechanical action of endodontic instruments requires another important characteristic of the auxiliary substances, which is to keep the walls of the root canal lubricated and hydrated, facilitating delivery and minimising friction on the walls of the root canal. This is later complemented by preparation of the canal using manual or rotational instrumentation to achieve the final filling (WEBER et al., 2003).

Sodium hypochlorite

In 1917, Barret disseminated the use of Dakin's solution for root canal irrigation and reported its efficiency as an antiseptic. Coolidge, in 1919, also used sodium hypochlorite to improve the root canal cleaning and disinfection process and, in 1936, Walker indicated the use of 5% sodium hypochlorite for preparing the root canals of teeth with necrotic pulps, as it helped to decontaminate the instruments, manipulate the root canals and protect the patient and operator, due to the microorganisms that a root canal can harbour (ESTEVES; FROES, 2013).

NaOCL is used in endodontics worldwide thanks to its behaviour as an SQA, mainly due to its efficacy in pulp dissolution and antimicrobial activity. A less concentrated solution, such as 1% sodium hypochlorite, has acceptable biological compatibility, although other authors recommend using higher concentrations (VARISE et al., 2014).

The irrigation of infected root canals is an important factor in the success of endodontic therapy. Sodium hypochlorite is a well-studied irrigant due to its antimicrobial effect, ability to dissolve tissue and acceptable biological compatibility at low concentrations. Accidents with sodium hypochlorite can occur when the irrigant comes into contact with periapical tissue or other soft tissues, which leads to severe inflammation (SALUM et al., 2012; VARISE et al., 2014; WEBER et al., 2003; WANG et al., 2010).

A current problem for endodontic clinicians is the extrusion of contaminated debris through the apical foramen. This phenomenon, known as flare-up, is responsible for causing headaches for endodontists. Professionals must therefore employ appropriate measures in an attempt to prevent serious flare-ups from occurring and must be able to treat them efficiently. One of the causes of **flare-up** may be the accidental extrusion of NaOCl into the periapical region, causing unpleasant events during treatment (SALUM et al., 2012; WANG et al., 2010; SÓ et al., 2011).

Table 2 - Comparison of the advantages and disadvantages of sodium hypochlorite.

Advantages	**Disadvantages**
Low cost	Unstable in storage
Fast action	Inactivated by organic matter
Deodorant and lubricant	Corrosive
Antimicrobial activity (bacteria, fungi and viruses)	Irritating to skin and mucous membranes
Non-toxic at appropriate concentrations	Strong odour
Solvent action of organic matter	Discolours fabrics
Easily determined concentrations	Removes carbon from rubber
Whitening	

Source: Salum et al., 2012.

Mechanism of action

Sodium hypochlorite, due to its high pH, is attributed its main antimicrobial characteristic, as it alters the structure of the cytoplasmic membrane and produces changes in cell metabolism. By exerting its proteolytic action, tissue dissolution and the dissolution rate of sodium hypochlorite are directly proportional to its concentration (ALTAMIRIANO et al., 2017).

Scheme 1. Saponification reaction.

$$R-\overset{\overset{O}{\|}}{C}-O-R + NaOH \rightarrow R-\overset{\overset{O}{\|}}{C}-O-Na + R-OH$$

Fatty acid | Sodium hydroxide | Soap | Glycerol

Scheme 2. Amino acid neutralization reaction.

$$R-\underset{\underset{NH_2}{|}}{\overset{\overset{H}{|}}{C}}-O-\overset{\overset{O}{//}}{\underset{OH}{C}} + NaOH \rightarrow R-\underset{\underset{NH_2}{|}}{\overset{\overset{H}{|}}{C}}-O-\overset{\overset{O}{//}}{\underset{ONa}{C}} + H_2O$$

Amino acid | Sodium hydroxide | Salt | Water

Scheme 3. Chloramination reaction.

$$R-\underset{\underset{NH_2}{|}}{\overset{\overset{H}{|}}{C}}-O-\overset{\overset{O}{//}}{\underset{OH}{C}} + HOCl \rightarrow R-\underset{\underset{NH_2}{|}}{\overset{\overset{Cl}{|}}{C}}-O-\overset{\overset{O}{//}}{\underset{OH}{C}} + H_2O$$

Amino acid | Hypochlorous acid | Chloramine | Water

Figure 12 - Chemical reactions of sodium hypochlorite with organic tissue.

Source: Estrela, 2002.

According to Estrela et al. (2002) these reactions (Figure 4) can be interpreted chemically by observing that sodium hypochlorite acts as an organic and fatty solvent, degrading fatty acids, generating fatty acid salts (soap) and glycerol (alcohol), reducing the surface tension of the residual solution (diagram 1). - saponification reaction. Sodium hypochlorite neutralises the amino acids, producing water and salt (diagram 2 - neutralisation reaction). When the hydroxyl ions leave, the pH decreases, making the environment more neutral. Hypochlorous acid, a substance present in sodium hypochlorite solution, when in contact with organic tissue acts as a solvent, releasing chlorine which, when combined with the amino group of the protein, forms chloramines (diagram 3 – chloramination reaction). Hypochlorous acid (HOCl-) and hypochlorite ions (OCl-) lead to the degradation and hydrolysis of amino acids.

Concentrations

As mentioned above, sodium hypochlorite can be **found in various concentrations. The concentration considered "safe"** can vary according to the authors and in endodontic treatment, as can be seen in Table 3. The antimicrobial property is proportional to the concentration of the drug, as is its toxicity (ALTAMIRIANO et al., 2017; CÁRDENAS et al., 2012).

Table 3 - NaOCl solutions in their different concentrations.

Name	C aracteristics
Dakin's liquid	0.5% sodium hypochlorite solution, neutralised with boric acid
Dausfrene liquid	0.5% sodium hypochlorite solution neutralised with sodium bicarbonate
Xilton's solution	1.0% sodium hypochlorite solution stabilised by sodium chloride (16%)
Labarraque liqueur	2.5% sodium hypochlorite solution
Chlorinated soda	Sodium hypochlorite solution of varying concentration between 4 and 6%
Sanitary water	2-2.5% sodium hypochlorite solutions

Source: Cárdenas et al., 2012.

Source: Cárdenas et al., 2012.

Adverse reactions

Chlorine (Cl2) is popularly the most common disinfectant used in water treatment, as it is easy to use and has effective germicidal properties at a low cost (FARREM et al., 2008). However, despite its antimicrobial effect, chlorine also reacts with dissolved organic material and produces disinfection by-products such as trihalomethanes (chloroform) and haloacetic acids. Daily exposure to chlorinated water can be hazardous to human health due to the carcinogenic and mutagenic properties of these compounds. The consumption of chlorinated products has been correlated with cancer risks (ESTRELA et al., 2002)

Sodium hypochlorite does not differentiate between vital and necrotic tissue, compromising the tissues surrounding the tooth. In addition, another disadvantage of hypochlorite is the corrosion of metal instruments. Several **in vitro** and **in vivo** studies have shown that this compound (NaOCL) is unable to remove the smear layer or the entire intra-root microbiota. It is therefore recommended to use this solution in conjunction with other compounds, such as chlorhexidine digluconate (FARREM et al., 2008; GERNHARDT et al., 2004).

Chlorhexidine digluconate

Chlorhexidine, also known as chlorhexidine digluconate, is a cationic bisbiguanide with both hydrophilic and hydrophobic properties, whose symmetrical molecule has two 4-chloro phenyl rings and two ethane pentane groups, linked by a central hexamethylene chain, and is chemically classified as chlorhexidine digluconate. It is generally more effective against Gram-positive micro-organisms than Gram-negative ones. Chlorhexidine is one of the antimicrobial agents widely used in mouthwashes, serving as the **gold standard** in antimicrobial activity studies (MACÊDO-COSTA; SANTOS et al., 2018).

Mechanism of action

DCLX is strongly absorbed by oral surfaces, being gradually released from the sites of action (substantivity) (MACÊDO-COSTA et al., 2018); it can reduce the growth and metabolism of dental biofilm, and the adherence potential of colonising microorganisms. It acts on the general disorganisation of the cell membrane and specific inhibition of membrane enzymes and inhibits the incorporation of glucose by **Streptococcus mutans** and its metabolism to lactic acid, and reduces the proteolytic activity of **Porphyromonas gingivalis** (DORNELLES et al., 2011).

As previously mentioned, the effect of DCLX is unquestionable and it is considered the gold standard in microbiological studies and in its clinical therapeutic application. However, continuous use of this substance causes some undesirable effects such as an unpleasant taste, staining of teeth and restorations, pigmentation of the tongue and flaking or damage to the oral mucosa (DORNELLES et al., 2011; GERBARA et al., 1996).

DCLX has a broad spectrum of action and can target Gram-positive and Gram-negative bacteria, yeasts and lipophilic viruses. Depending on its concentration, its effect can be bactericidal or bacteriostatic. At high concentrations, its effect is bactericidal, as it breaks down the cell wall, interfering with transport and also interfering with coagulation in the cytoplasm due to its high affinity with the protein.

At low concentrations, it has a bacteriostatic action, inhibiting membrane function, and its effect is maintained for several hours after its application (YAMASHITA et al., 2013; MICHELOTTO et al., 2008; ALMEIDA et al., 2014).

Concentrations

DCLX is commercially available in various forms of presentation and concentration. These include: lotion, ointment, gel or in the form of disinfectant soap. This substance is used in dentistry for clinical application in various procedures, with varying presentations and concentrations, ranging from 0.2% to 2.0%. The 2% concentration, used in Endodontics, comes in gel or liquid form and is colourless, slightly opalescent, odourless or almost odourless, its taste is usually bitter and can be masked in formulations intended for oral use. The unpleasant flavour and taste interference of chlorhexidine are considered undesirable effects (ALMEIDA et al., 2014; ALTAMIRIANO et al., 2017; SURESHCHANDRA et al., 2011).

Adverse reactions

As already mentioned in the previous topic, chlorhexidine has side effects, such as: temporal sensation of interference in the taste of food, stains on teeth, dentures and tongue surface (GUNESER et al., 2016). According to Altamiriano et al. (2017), the use of chlorhexidine on oral microorganisms and human gingival fibroblasts shows moderate cytotoxic effects on cellular components.

DCLX is often credited with being less damaging and more biocompatible than sodium hypochlorite in all its concentrations. In order to test the tissue inflammatory response to irrigating agents, Yamashita et al. (2013) carried out an in vivo study. The results showed that 2% chlorhexidine did not induce a significant inflammatory response and was similar to the control used, unlike 0.5% sodium hypochlorite (GUNESER et al., 2016).

CHAPTER 6

HERBAL MEDICINES AND THE USE OF PLANT EXTRACTS IN ENDODONTICS

CARLUS ALBERTO OLIVEIRA DOS SANTOS;
KAROLYNE DE MELO SOARES;
MARIA REGINA MACÊDO-COSTA.

A herbal medicine is defined as a plant extract or preparation containing crude or processed ingredients from one or more plants with therapeutic values (SURESHCHANDRA et al., 2011). Due to safety concerns, side effects, a steady increase in antibiotic resistance and the ineffectiveness of conventional drug formulations, researchers are interested in herbal alternatives that have been widely used in medical practice for many centuries and have become even more popular today due to their biocompatibility, anti-inflammatory properties, antimicrobial properties, antioxidant properties and less toxicity and antimicrobial resistance problems (GUPTA et al., 2015; MACÊDO-COSTA et al., 2018; ALAGL et al., 2017).

Decontamination is achieved during the chemical surgical preparation of the root canal, in which mechanical cleaning enables prophylaxis and modelling of the main canal, while chemical cleaning reaches areas not affected by instrumentation, such as the branches of the main canal and the apical region (DI SANTI et al., 2015). This chemical action is represented by the use of irrigating solutions and intracanal medication. These bacteria are able to invade and remain viable inside dentinal tubules for a prolonged period of time, adhere and form biofilm on dentin under different environmental conditions, resist intracanal disinfectants, and survive in adverse conditions in filled root canals (ROCHA et al., 2013; GONZALES et al., 2017).

Intracanal antimicrobial medicaments are used to complement the disinfection of the root canal system. Calcium hydroxide is widely used due to its biological properties and antimicrobial activity, inhibiting tooth resorption and inducing hard tissue formation, stimulating osteoblast proliferation, and its ability to inactivate bacterial endotoxins (VASCONCELOS, 2016; DI SANTI et al., 2015).

Plant essential oils have been used since the dawn of human civilisation for therapeutic and medicinal purposes. Melaleuca oil (OM) promotes lysis and loss of cell membrane integrity and function, manifested by ion leakage and inhibition of respiration. This compound has been shown to be effective against 15 strains of MRSA and 5 strains of vancomycin-resistant enterococci (VASCONCELOS, 2016; MACÊDO- COSTA; SANTOS et al., 2018; ALAGL et al., 2017).

Curcumin, a member of the ginger family, has been widely publicised as having anti-inflammatory, antioxidant, antimicrobial and anticancer activity. **In vitro** studies have revealed that curcumin has remarkable antibacterial action against **E. faecalis** and can be used as a substitute for NaOCl for endodontic irrigations (ALAGL et al., 2017; SURESHCHANDRA et al., 2011).

Table 4 - Plant extracts active on **Enterococcus faecalis.**

Sl.No.	Scientific Name	Common name	Pharmacological active ingredients	Extract type	References
1	*Curcuma longa*	Saffron Indian saffron yellow ginger	Zingiberene. curcumin. a and (J turmerone	Ethyl acetate, methanol and water extracts	Marickar et al Neelakantan etal
2	*Propolis*	Beeswax	Flavonoids Aromatic acids Esters present in resins. Galangin Pinocebrin	Ethanol, chloroform, methanol, propylene glycol	Oncag O et al Al-Qathami H et al Kandaswamy etal
3	*Aloe vera*	Star cactus, bearded	Glucomannan latex, mannose derivatives. hemicellulose. calcium oxalate	Aqueous, ethanol and methanolic extracts	George et al Karkare etal. Sureshchandra et al
4	*Azadiracnta indica*	Neem. sacred tree	Azadirachtin nimbin gallic acid catechin	Aqueous, ethanol, chloroform and methanolic extracts of seeds, leaves, fruit and roots	Nayak et al
5	*Monnda w/tnfolia*	Indian mulberry, analgesic shrub, fruit of	L-asperuloid. acubin. alantin kaempferol acid	Aqueous extracts. Ethanol and methanol	Murrayetal, Prabhakar et al

Source: Alagl, 2017

Genus Spondias

According to Silva et al. (2014), Anacardiaceae is a plant family made up of approximately 60-75 genera and around 600 species. These species are distributed in tropical, subtropical and temperate zones, the prototype of the Brazilian semi-arid region. The genus is known for its economic importance and pharmaceutical properties thanks to its phytoconstituents or active ingredients. Spondias, for example, is a tropical genus of this family with 14 to 20 species distributed worldwide, and of these,

4 to 7 species are found in the Americas, especially South America.

In Brazil, among the species of the genus Spondias, we can highlight the commercial importance of cajá (**S. mombin**), umbu (**S. tuberosa**) and cajá-umbu (**S. mombin x S. tuberosa**). The fruit is sold fresh or processed into pulp, juice and other food products. Due to the commercial use of these fruits, studies have looked into their cultivation characteristics, as well as their physicochemical characteristics, ripeness and stability, and chemical constituents (NJOKU et al., 2007; SEERAM et al., 2005; DELPRETE et al., 2014).

Spondias mombin

Cajá (**Spondias mombin**) is a small, elliptical fruit 3-4 cm long, grown in the north-east of Brazil. Its commercial use has increased in recent years due to its accessibility, year-round availability and easy preparation. As an example, the fruits of the cajazeira (**S. mombin**) are used as frozen pulps and pasteurised juices (SEERAM et al., 2005; SILVA et al., 2014).

As previously mentioned, **Spondias Monbim,** popularly **known as "cajá", belongs to the** Anacardiaceae family **and** is found in countries such as Peru, Brazil, Venezuela, Bolivia, Colombia, the Three Guianas, as well as southern Mexico, Belize, Costa Rica and the Antilles (ALMEIDA et al., 2011). The leaves are used to gargle, as an astringent, in inflammations of the mouth and throat. There are reports of its use in the mouth in cases of prostatitis and cold sores. With regard to biological activities, the following have been cited: antimicrobial activity (SILVA et al., 2014).

Research using the methanolic extract of cajazeira (**S. mombin**) leaves showed antibacterial activity against Pseudomonas aeruginosa and Shigella dysenteriae, while extracts of the stem bark inhibited the growth of Escherichia coli and Klebsiella pneumoniae bacteria. Although the extracts do not show significant antifungal activity, some antimicrobial activity is attributed to the presence of tannins, saponins and anthraquinones (ABO et al., 1999; ALBUQUERQUE et al., 2007).

Antimicrobial activity of Spondias mombin

The proven antimicrobial effect of the cajá extract is due to the presence of the anarcadic acid derivative, isolated from the leaves of the cajazeira tree (**S.** *mombin),* **which has the ability to inhibit the action of** 0-lactamase, an activity also attributed to clavulanic acid, a commercially known antibacterial (COATES et al., 1994).

In addition to the antibacterial and antiviral activities proven in laboratory tests, other antibiotic activities are attributed to extracts of cajazeira (**S. mombin**) leaves. Antifungal activity is used in traditional African medicine, but its laboratory evidence is still controversial, with studies referring to weak activity on strains of filamentous fungi and yeasts, and others in which no antifungal activity was found (ABO et al., 1999; SEERAM et al., 2005).

The results showed the presence of some secondary metabolites, including phenolic compounds, flavonoids, tannins and saponins, in agreement with what was found by Silva et al. (2013) and Corthout et al. (1992) in their study.

Given that several studies have proven the effectiveness of phenolic compounds, flavonoids and tannins as antimicrobial and antioxidant agents, it can be suggested that the great antibacterial activity shown by **S. mombin** is due to the presence of these metabolites in its composition (ELZAAWELY et al., 2005; CORTHOUT et al., 1994).

The presence of ellagic acid and quercetin was also noted. The presence of these metabolites in the **S. mombin** extract has already been reported by Silva et al. (2012), who believe that their existence guarantees the extract its antibacterial and antioxidant activities.

As well as having antibacterial activity, the literature reports that quercetin exhibits antioxidant activity, DNA protection activity and anti-humour effect, while ellagic acid has antioxidant, anticancer, antimutagenic and antiproliferative activities (SEERAM et al., 2005; LOARCA- PINA et al., 1998; REN et al., 2003; WHITLEY et al., 2013; CUSHINE; LAMB, 2005).

Spondias Tuberosa

Spondias tuberosa, or umbu, is a tree species that is important both as an economic resource and as an alternative livelihood for rural communities in the semi-arid regions of northeastern Brazil (NETO et al., 2010).

This plant has phenolic compounds, which suggest promising antimicrobial pharmacological potential. However, studies proving this action against microbial isolates of clinical origin are still scarce. (ALBUQUERQUE et al., 2016)

Intracanal medication and the use of natural products

Decontamination is achieved during the chemical surgical preparation of the root canal, in which mechanical cleaning enables prophylaxis and modelling of the main canal, while chemical cleaning reaches areas not affected by instrumentation, such as the branches of the main canal and the apical region. This chemical action is represented by the use of irrigating solutions and intracanal medication. These bacteria are capable of invading and remaining viable inside dentinal tubules for a prolonged period of time, adhering and forming biofilm on dentin under different environmental conditions, resisting intracanal disinfectants and surviving under adverse conditions in filled root canals (ROCHA et al., 2013).

Intracanal antimicrobial medicaments are used to complement the disinfection of the root canal system. Calcium hydroxide is widely used due to its biological properties and antimicrobial activity, inhibiting tooth resorption and inducing hard tissue formation, stimulating osteoblast proliferation, and its ability to inactivate bacterial endotoxins (VASCONCELOS, 2016; DI SANTI et al., 2015).

Plant essential oils have been used since the dawn of human civilisation for therapeutic and medicinal purposes. Melaleuca oil (OM) promotes lysis and loss of cell membrane integrity and function, manifested by ion leakage and inhibition of respiration. This compound proved effective against 15 strains of MRSA and 5 strains of vancomycin-resistant enterococci (VASCONCELOS, 2016).

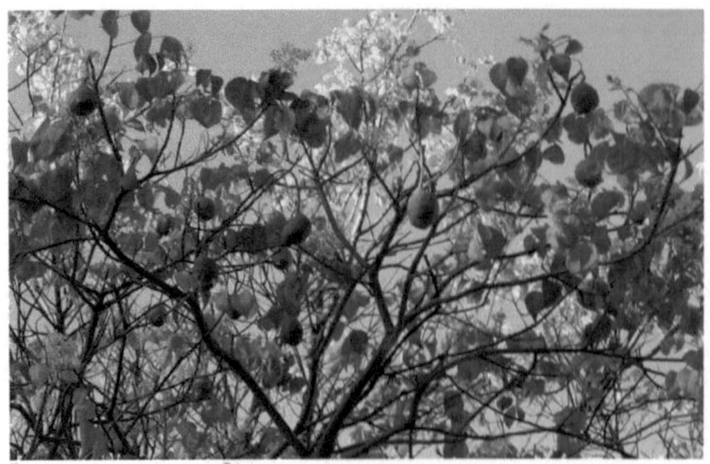

Figure 12: Cajaz tree with green cajá fruit.
Source: Natureza bela, 2011

Genus Genipa L.

According to Delprete, Smith and Klein (2004), **Genipa** L. has been recognised as a genus with only two species: **G. americana** L. **and G. infundibuliformis Zappi & Semir.** The first is native and cultivated throughout the Neotropics, from Mexico to Patagonia, and the second species has so far only been found in central and southern Brazil.

The leaves are opposite and crossed, with petioles. The inflorescences are axillary or terminal, with five or six flowers arranged at the base and are usually hermaphrodite. The fruit is a simple berry, subglobose, oblong or obovoid in shape with many seeds (SOBBEN et al., 2003; MOURA et al., 2016;).

This genus has several uses, such as as edible fruit, used to prepare juices, jellies and liqueurs. The indigenous tribes of South America use the fruit to dye fabrics, hammocks, wooden utensils and their bodies. The wood is used in carpentry and the bark, rich in tannin, is used in tanneries to treat hides. As a medicinal plant it is indicated as a diuretic, antifebrile, for the treatment of external wounds and pharyngitis (SOBBEN et al., 2003; VIEIRA et al., 2006).

Genipa americana **L.**

Riparian forests are an important ecosystem whose main function is to preserve river banks, preventing erosion and consequent silting, as well as providing food for aquatic fauna. These forests play a strategic role in conserving biodiversity, preserving water quality and forming genetic corridors between the few primary forests that exist on river banks (SOBBEN et al., 2003; VIEIRA et al., 2006).

It is a natural vegetation component in the dense ombrophilous forest region of the Atlantic slope in southern Brazil, in the Paraná River Basin and in the state of Paraná. The species is native to Neotropical countries, but its exact origin is not known. There are reports of its use by indigenous Tupi-Guarani tribes native to the Americas (COSTA et al., 2005; MOREIRA et al 2002).

The species, known as jenipapo, is a tree-like plant with the characteristics of a selective hygrophyte and is considered to be of great ecological and economic importance, both for its use in mixed plantations in degraded permanent preservation areas and for food production. Several chemical substances were identified in the **G. americana** species (figure 1), such as mannitol, tannins, methyl ethers, hydantoin, tannic acids and, above all, iridoids, which are characteristic of the family. Among the isolated glycoside iridoids. After surveying some of the plants found in the north-east of Brazil, it was reported that the infusion of leaves is used against liver diseases and the fruit is considered a tonic against anaemia. A community in Ilhéus, Bahia, uses the fruit as a syrup and/or juice for anaemia and coughs (MOURA et al. 2016; ANDRADE et al., 2000; VALERI et al., 2003).

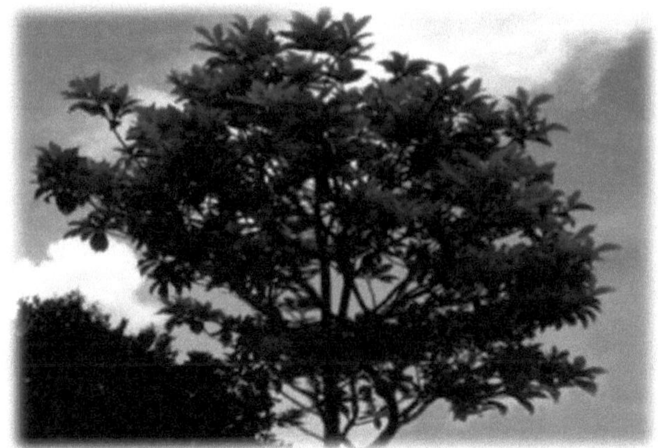

Figure 13: Tree of the species **G. americana** L.

Source: Moreira et al, 2002.

Discussion

As previously reported, plants are an excellent source for finding new antimicrobial drugs, given that the molecular diversity of natural products is much greater than that derived from chemical synthesis processes. Although research using plants as an alternative for treating mouth ailments is relatively recent, empirical application is quite old.

The low cost of herbal medicines, making them more accessible to the population, thanks to the possibility of them having fewer side effects or toxic effects, like sodium hypochlorite, and their wide acceptance by the population (SILVA et al., 2011).

The antimicrobial activity of plant extracts comes from the presence of some secondary metabolites, including phenolic compounds, flavonoids, tannins and saponins, in agreement with what was found by Silva et al. (2012) and Corthout et al. (1992). Various studies have proven the effectiveness of phenolic compounds, flavonoids and tannins as antimicrobial and antioxidant agents (NASCIMENTO et al., 2000; ELZAAWELY et al., 2005; CORTHOUT et al., 1994).

Like conventional antimicrobial agents, not all extracts are effective against all MOs, especially when it comes to superinfecting MOs or those related to persistent infections. According to Viera et al. (2006), these MOs include **Enterococcus faecalis and Staphylococcus aureus,** known for their potential for microbial resistance.

Costa et al., (2008) states that in dentistry, the presence of **Enterococcus faecalis** inside canals has been associated with persistent endodontic infections, which has led to the development of research to evaluate the effectiveness of the antimicrobial action of intracanal medicines and irrigating solutions.

Several comparative studies have been carried out using substances already used clinically as controls, such as sodium hypochlorite and chlorhexidine digluconate. Although sodium hypochlorite is used worldwide because of its excellent antimicrobial action, it has some limitations when it comes to multi-resistant microbial species, such as **S. aureus.**

In addition to its antimicrobial capacity, one of the main advantages that justifies the use of sodium hypochlorite-based solutions in endodontics is their ability to dissolve organic tissue, which is not observed with chlorhexidine (LEONARDO et al., 1999).

Concluding their study, Leonardo et al. (1999) stated that chlorhexidine performed best, followed by calcium hydroxide, propolis extract and finally 5% sodium hypochlorite.

Although the level of reliability of in vitro studies is validated, other factors can influence the results obtained. Altamiriano et al. (2017) explains that the geographical location where the extracts were obtained, as well as how the substances were stored and the means of production influence the interpretation of the results.

Sodium hypochlorite, for example, is an agent with considerable chemical instability, and even the way it is stored can negatively influence its antimicrobial capacity. These problems can be circumvented when the material tested follows a strict selection protocol (WERLANG et al., 2016).

Antimicrobial activity is just one of the desirable requirements of SQAs, as well as helping to debride the root canal system, having the ability to dissolve organic tissue, exhibiting good lubricating capacity, offering surface tension in order to access inaccessible areas, preventing the formation of smearlayer during instrumentation and not having cytotoxic effects on periradicular tissues. Therefore, other capacities should be evaluated in plant extracts, not just microbiological studies (LERONARDO et al., 1999; SIQUEIRA JUNIOR et al., 2001; MACÊDO-COSTA; SANTOS et al., 2018).

With the limitations of the studies available in the literature, more laboratory and clinical research is needed to evaluate the safety, efficacy and biocompatibility of other plant extracts before finally recommending them as alternative endodontic irrigants. Finally, clinically tested plant extracts should only be used for established treatment procedures (UNDERGER et al., 2004)

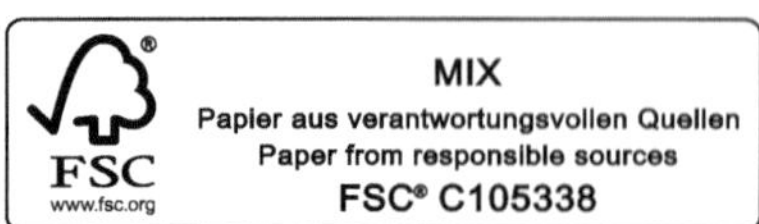

Printed by Books on Demand GmbH, Norderstedt / Germany